Miracle in My Arms

PRAYERS FOR A NEW MOTHER

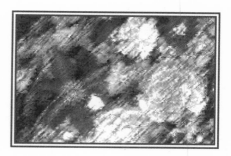

Shelley Swanson Sateren

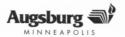

Augsburg
MINNEAPOLIS

MIRACLE IN MY ARMS
Prayers for a New Mother

Cover and interior design by Lois Stanfield, LightSource Images

Library of Congress Cataloging-in-Publication Data
Sateren, Shelley Swanson.
   Miracle in my arms : prayers for a new mother / by Shelley
  Swanson Sateren.
    p. cm.
   ISBN 0-8066-2726-3
   1. Mothers—Prayer-books and devotions—English. 2. Pregnant
  women—Prayer-books and devotions—English. I. Title.
BV4847.S28 1995
242'.8431—dc20   95-40338
                                                                CIP

Manufactured in the U.S.A.   AF 9-2726

99 98 97 96 95 1 2 3 4 5 6 7 8 9 10

To Erik, my son and beloved treasure,
and
To Roald, my husband and truelove.

Contents

Preface   9

This New Life   11
Miracle in My Arms   13
Frightening What Ifs   15
Heal the Hurts, Lord   18
This Wondrous Being   21
New Angel Assignments   22

Beloved Newcomer   25
Fragile—Handle with Care   27
Who's the Baby Here?   29
A Bad Case of the Inadequacies   33
Tiny Infant = Giant Impact   36
My Good Fortune   41
The Bitter Cup of Colic   45
Heaven-sent Baby Shower Presents   51

Feeling His Pain   55
Spreading Sunshine   57

Post-Baby Family Life   59
Fearing an Untimely Good-bye   61
Routines in Ruins   63
No Other Mother Knows   68
Uproot the Bitter-fruit Tree, Lord   70
Clashes in Wedlock   73
Busy Baby, Busy Days   78
A Momentous First: Missed!   81
Half Birthday, Wholly Thankful   85
Center of My Universe   89

New Challenges   91
Yet a Freshman Mother   93
The Load of Adulthood   96
Longer Trips to Dreamland   99
Unblemished Babies   101
A Wellspring of Joy   104
Irretrievable Babyhood   108

Angels to My Aid   111

A Houseful of Germs   113

Saying No   116

Our Dear Child, Already Ruined   122

Visit from an Angel   124

Sunnier Days   127

A New Means of Locomotion   130

Happy Birthday!   133

Safeguard Our Beloved Child   137

Simply Because a Mother Asks   139

Social Trials   144

Home Improvements   147

As a Boy and as a Man   151

The Best Defense   155

This Gift from Heaven   158

Preface

My first year as a new mother was simultaneously the most pain-filled and joy-filled year I've ever known. During those turbulent weeks and months after my baby's birth, I wished I'd had a book on my nightstand to help me spiritually as well as emotionally.

This collection sprang out of that wish.

From the outset of my labor pains through the spectacular first birthday party a year later, I wrote about my feelings in a quickly-scribbled journal and prayed often. Prayer became a powerful means of transcending my difficulties—and affirming my delight—as an overwhelmed and overjoyed new mother.

May this collection provide for other new mothers the bedside companion I yearned for during my first year with my baby. God bless you and your family during your first year with your new baby and as your family grows up together.

This New Life

Miracle in My Arms

Oh thank you, God!
for the passing of the labor pain,
for replacing the pain with rapture,
for the overpowering love I'm feeling
for this new little person.

Thank you, God!
for sparing him,
for sparing me,
for preserving us both from the dangers of childbirth.

Thank you, God!
for listening to my nine-month-long plea:
for giving us a healthy baby—a huge relief to my
husband and me,
for granting us even more than we asked for—
a beautiful baby, when all we hoped for was a
       healthy child.

Thank you, God!
for this sunrise that's casting radiance on this new day,
this new life,
for filling my heart to near-bursting with the purest
        love
I've ever known,
for this beautiful little miracle lying in my arms.

Frightening What Ifs

I'm alone in my hospital bed, Lord,
the afternoon of my baby's birth,
and the excitement is dying down.
Sheer exhaustion is taking over
and I'm starting to experience aftershocks.
I'm trembling and teary now, in recollecting
the difficult labor that I had to endure.
I've never worked so hard, been so exhausted,
or experienced such pain in my life—
and I believe with conviction that no pain
in my future will ever compare.
I had little fear of my forthcoming labor during my
          pregnancy,
but now that it's over, now that I know what labor's
          like,
(at least for me anyway; I know it's easier for some
          mothers),

I'm scared after the fact, Lord—
scared for myself,
scared for my baby,
as my mind uncontrollably entertains frightening
        What Ifs.
No doubt this terrible fatigue and hormonal upheaval
I'm feeling today are contributing to this anxious state.
Please, Lord, comfort me.

I'm scared today, God, considering the possibility
that my baby's birth could have been even worse.
What if I'd lived one hundred years ago?
What if I lived in a country with poor medical
        facilities?
I might not have survived
and very likely my baby wouldn't have lived.
I am so thankful, Lord, and yet my heart aches
for the women and babies throughout the world
        today
who don't have access to decent medical services.
For these women and their babies,
the frightening What Ifs become horrific reality.
I pray for these women and their babies, Lord.
Please protect their miracles.

I also pray, Lord,
for mothers who have had difficult labors
and whose babies have survived,
yet who later discover their babies were disabled
by the trauma of their difficult births.
Please, Lord, ease these mothers' despair
and their babies' suffering.

Heal the Hurts, Lord

My baby is one and a half days old now, Lord,
and I'm sending up a plea for his speedy recovery.
He's noticeably marred from the birth journey,
the most difficult trip he'll ever take in his life.
His head has open sores from the electrodes,
has a large, purple, puffy bruise from the vacuum
        suction,
and is misshapen from maneuvering down the narrow
        canal.
My baby's also struggling to adjust to life outside the
        womb,
choking on mucous as he tries to breathe oxygen,
working hard as he learns to nurse from my breasts,
and now, suffering from this morning's circumcision.
I'm sorry for any and all ways that I've
contributed to his discomfort, Lord,
since it was my body that caused a difficult birth
        for him,

and it was my husband's and my decision to have him
      circumcised.
I'm heartsick seeing my tiny, helpless baby hurting so.
Please, Lord, help him heal swiftly.

I'm sending up another plea today, Lord,
for my husband's recuperation.
A day and a half following our baby's birth,
my husband is still emotionally shaken
from having witnessed my painful labor,
still physically exhausted from loss of sleep,
still wrung out from having worked and worried
      very hard
as my doting and dutiful coach,
still troubled by the memories of our baby's
distress signals on the monitor
and from seeing the midwife and surgeon's concerned
      faces,
and from watching me writhe in pain for hours on end.
Please, Lord, quicken my husband's recovery.

I'm sending up a third plea today, Lord,
for the final member of our small family—me.
A day and a half after my baby's birth,

I'm sobbing as I sit here in my sitz bath,
crying from fatigue and physical discomfort
in the aftermath of my labor—
the marathon of a lifetime!
And now my hormones are having a heyday,
and to top it off, I'm feeling overcome by the
    avalanche
of baby-care and mommy-care details
distributed by the nurses, doctors, and midwives.
Please, Lord, steady me soon
and quickly restore me.

ॐ

This Wondrous Being

It's two o'clock in the morning, Lord,
and in the dim light of this hospital room
my nearly two-day-old baby is quietly nursing
and I'm awestruck yet again at the sight
of his perfect, minute ears and nose and cheeks and chin.
I'm mesmerized as I gaze upon this blinking, breathing
      marvel—
this new little life which belongs to me.
Dear God, I know the creation
of this tiny, extraordinary creature
was your wonderwork.
I'm wholly grateful to you, Lord,
for the gift of this wondrous being,
      this baby.

New Angel Assignments

Our baby is two and a half days old now, Lord,
and it's time to take him home.
We're all packed and ready to leave the hospital,
but even before we've left the safe confines
of this medical building,
I've already spied two things in the parking lot
that could cause harm to our vulnerable new baby—
a cloud of exhaust billowing out of a car
and a speeding taxi.

It's time to ask you, God, on behalf of our baby,
that you grant him his own guardian angel,
an ever-present, protective companion,
to guide him, watch over him, comfort him, provide
     for him,
and shield him from all possible harm on the horizon—
today, tomorrow, and throughout his days on Earth.

Also, dear Lord,
my husband's new role as the father
and my new role as the mother
of this vulnerable infant
require, it seems, new angel assignments.
Please grant each of us a personal angel,
so that this new mommy
and this new daddy
are guided and protected throughout our little one's
    childhood,
during the years when he would be lost without
    loving parents.

Beloved
Newcomer

❧

Fragile—Handle with Care

Our beloved little newcomer
has been home for only six hours, Lord,
and I'm already frightened silly.
Just look at me!
I'm creeping down these steps at a snail's pace,
carrying in my arms this living, breathing, priceless
        package
with invisible letters written all over him:
FRAGILE—HANDLE WITH CARE.
What's to stop me from taking a misguided step
on these slippery stairs,
and toppling down the stairwell
and catapulting my completely defenseless baby out of
        my arms?
I just can't protect my tiny, breakable baby entirely on
        my own.
I pray for your help in watching over him, dear Lord.

Please forgive my weak faith, God, if in the months to
        come
I send up frequent pleas
asking that you tend to my baby's health and safety.
Please remind me that our dear child
and his mommy and daddy
are all in your constant care.
And please continue to guide my feet
on these deadly hardwood stairs.

Who's the Baby Here?

These first postpartum days have been so hard on me,
    Lord.
I'm tired, I'm weary, I'm weepy.
I hurt in both body and spirit.
During this first week with our new baby,
I feel like a baby in need of babying too.
I wish someone would gather me up in his or her
        arms
and dry my tears,
then lower me into a drawn bubble bath,
then lay me down on my bed and pull a blanket up
        to my chin,
and reassure me that everything will be fine.
But wishing is fruitless, I know.
There's no one to baby me
the way I wish to be babied this week—

not my mother,
not my husband,
not even myself.

Not since my childhood days have I felt the need
to be showered with mother love
the way I have this week, Lord.
Now that I'm a mommy it seems I've unexpectedly
     regressed
and need my own "mommy" more than ever.
Some of the sadness I'm feeling this week
is due, I believe, to grieving.
When I gave birth,
the final flickerings of my own childhood died out,
and I'm mourning that loss, Lord.
My mother can never again cradle me in her arms
and comfort me when I'm sad or mad or hurt
the way she did when I was a tiny girl.
It's my turn to do that for my baby;
I'm the parent now.

My husband's a parent now too.
I used to be his "babe" but now he's got a new babe,
and he's giving his new baby all he's got.

That doesn't leave a whole lot left over for me, Lord.
My husband's much too busy babying our new baby
to baby me anymore.
The two of us used to talk baby talk to each other,
privately, intimately,
but suddenly that's ceased too.
All gibberish is now reserved for the new baby of the
        house.
I miss my husband's and my baby talk very much,
but our new grown-up roles don't seem to allow it,
at least not right now.

Even I am incapable of babying myself
the way I long to be babied today, Lord.
Nearly all of my energy is being consumed
in caring for our little newcomer.
I'm too tired and too busy to adequately care for
        myself.
I'm not resting enough, exercising enough,
or eating enough healthy food.
And I'm not asking for help
with child care when I need it;
I've always had trouble asking others for assistance . . .
except from you, Lord.

I know I can always come to you
and freely ask you for your help.
Please comfort me and support me.
I need your love desperately today.
Thank you for cradling me in your arms, Lord.

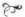

A Bad Case
of the Inadequacies

The second week at home with our baby has begun,
    Lord,
and I've developed a bad case of the Inadequacies.

I'm afraid I'm not responsible enough, Lord.
Never before have I had this degree of responsibility
    in any job.
CEOs of major corporations aren't this accountable;
vulnerable little human lives aren't totally dependent
    on them
for nurturing and security
the way my baby is all-dependent on me.
It's also entirely up to me to nourish my child—
since I'm breastfeeding exclusively.
I don't know if I'm capable of a job of such
    consequence.

Sometimes I wonder if I'm being a good mama.
Please, God, instill confidence in me.

I'm afraid I'm not smart enough, Lord.
I'm feeling swamped by tidal waves of baby-care details,
and troubled because I don't have a clue
if I'm doing anything right.
I feel like a kindergartner attending Baby Care
     University;
everything is an infant-care research project,
such as our baby's extreme case of infant acne,
and the vacuum-suction-induced bruise on his head
that's filling with fluid,
and the numerous breastfeeding trials we're experiencing.
I feel so green
and I'm afraid I'll do something wrong.
Please, Lord, grant me some self-assurance soon.

I'm afraid I'm not strong enough, Lord.
I'm learning it takes the physical strength of Hercules
to pace a room for more than an hour,
trying to pacify a screaming infant who refuses to nap
and refuses to breastfeed,
when I myself have slept a grand total

of three hours of broken sleep the night before,
and I myself have had no time to eat
anything more than a couple of stale corn chips.
Dear God, I'm desperately tired,
and my energy stores are dangerously low
from these lingering postpartum blues
and from this round-the-clock infant care.
I want to collapse in a heap
and cry my eyes out.
Please, Lord, reenergize me and help me to carry on—
at least until my husband comes home.

I suppose these new-mommy inadequacies
are a mixed blessing, Lord.
If I felt that I could handle it all,
I wouldn't call the clinic with my list of questions,
I wouldn't consult the experts in books,
and most importantly, I wouldn't come to you.
If I didn't turn to you for help, Lord,
I'd really be in trouble.
I truly believe that.
Thank you for humility.

Tiny Infant = Giant Impact

After nine years, married life
had become pretty orderly and efficient and
        predictable,
as you know, Lord,
but after just nine days with our new baby
it seems everything has changed.
Everything is different now,
everything is topsy-turvy,
and out-of-control,
and entirely disorganized.
I never dreamed two lives and a whole home
could change so drastically so suddenly.
Some of our friends who have children tried to
        forewarn us,
but I didn't listen to them,
I didn't believe them.

Please, Lord, help calm this hurricane on the home
   front.

One unanticipated change has hit me especially hard,
   Lord:
I've had to readjust my expectations dramatically
because time is no longer mine.
In my life-before-baby I used to leap from room to
   room
and accomplish a million tasks in a twenty-four hour
   period.
But now my days are consumed by baby-care duties
so I can't eat when I want to,
I can't set out on a walk when I feel like it,
and I certainly can't sleep when I need to
since I'm sharing sleeping quarters with a human
   alarm clock
who demands a breastfeed nearly every two hours.
I know tending to my baby's needs is top priority,
   God,
but there's no denying that this fact is clashing
with my attitude from my "former life"
that I always needed to be accomplishing something.

I just can't seem to get anything done anymore, Lord,
except for baby-care tasks.
Please, God, remind me that caring for my baby
is accomplishing something extremely important.
And please help me to relax and simply enjoy
spending these precious moments with him.

Of all the unanticipated changes, the worst is this, Lord:
the sudden transformation in my marital relationship.
Overnight, it seems, we've become pitted against each
        other
and short-tempered with one another.
Our shifting roles and responsibilities,
our quadrupled workload,
and our extreme exhaustion from these sleepless nights
have left us easily upset
and have caused several voice raisings this week.
This terrible fatigue leads to terrible fights!
We're both stunned and saddened by this change, Lord.
It's particularly troubling because we were so romantic
and supportive of each other during our pregnancy.
Suddenly my husband and I seem to care little for each
        other
and care everything for our baby instead.

Never before in our pre-baby life together
was my husband ever so excited to come home from
        work.
Now he grabs his gurgling son the moment he steps
        in the door
and tunes his daddy-antennae completely to him.
Yesterday my husband returned from a day of playing
        golf
and gushed to our baby, "I thought about you *all*
        afternoon!"
He's never said that to *me* after a day away from
        home.
I do feel invisible, Lord, and it's painful.
I admit that I'm also guilty
of disregarding my husband's presence
in exactly the same way,
with my full attention almost constantly on our
brand-new baby.
Placing our concern for each other
on the back burner, it seems, is keeping
our once-boiling pot of romance just barely luke-
        warm now.
I know, Lord, the books, articles, and experts say
that my husband and I are in the majority;

they say that the quality of most marriages declines
after the birth of a first child.
But why do *we* have to be in the majority, Lord?
We both suddenly feel inadequate as spouses
because we're expending most of our energy
in trying to be good parents.
Dear Lord, please give my husband and me marital
    strength
in abundance during this stressful period of
    adjustment.

My Good Fortune

I looked into the mirror this morning, Lord,
and saw a raccoon.
I had round, black bags under my eyes
from yet another terrible night's sleep.
I'm afraid our baby is a catnapper both by day and by
     night.
But even when he does snooze for a short while in the
     night,
I'm not always able to
because of my painfully engorged breasts
and from these awful hot flashes that make me wake up
in a sea of sweaty sheets.

Through a thick fog of exhaustion,
I dragged myself and my baby
to his two-week pediatric checkup this morning, Lord.
My parents met us at the clinic, gave us a ride home,

then dropped us off on our doorstep
and drove on to the cabin for the weekend.
I felt unbearably lonely
when my parents left me this morning, Lord,
alone to care for my little one—
when I felt I could lie down and die from fatigue,
when I knew my baby wouldn't nap well all day,
when I knew he'd spend much of the day crying,
when I knew I'd have to dig deep in my reserves
for the strength to console him
when my husband was away for the day
and there was no one else to help me.
As I watched my parents' car pull away,
the tears began, Lord.

But now, *at last*, my husband's home,
and we agreed it might cheer me up
if I took the dog on a walk in the park—
my first walk with the dog since our baby's birth.
Leaving the house behind
and meandering beneath the pines in this lovely park
with the sun kissing the top of my head
the thick fog of fatigue is beginning to clear,
and I'm now seeing a startling sight for the first time:

my good fortune.
I'm sorry, God;
it seems all I've done for two full weeks is complain.
Yes, these first two weeks with our new baby
have been stressful and tiring,
but what if he hadn't been born healthy?
What if something had been wrong with him?
This sunshine-filled stroll through the park
is lifting my spirits, Lord,
and I'm suddenly aware of how richly you've blessed us.

Thank you, God, that our baby is healthy and thriving.
Thank you that he's growing more cutely plump
with each passing day.
Thank you for the sweet forgiveness
between my husband and me
after our disagreements this week.
Thank you for the blessed moments as I hold my baby
in my arms
and gaze into his slate-blue eyes,
when I forget everything but how dear and adorable
he is.
Thank you, Lord, that my husband and I
were able to conceive this child.

We're aware that many couples don't share this good
        fortune.
Please ease their sorrow, Lord.
And please remind me to be truly grateful
for this marvelous gift, our baby.

The Bitter Cup of Colic

Monday morning
Our two-and-a-half-week-old catnapper
slept little and screamed lots all weekend, Lord,
napping only in the tiniest of bits and pieces
both day and night,
and waking up from each brief sleep shrieking—
shrieks that curled all ten of my toes.
His crying spells grew more intense and more
    inconsolable,
and any tricks we tried—
even driving him around the neighborhood in the
    car—
wouldn't calm him for long.
By last night, if someone had touched me
with the tip of a feather,
I would've burst into tears.
Dear God, I'm tense from our baby's terrible
    screaming,

45

I'm weary from his too-short daytime naps
(which mean no breaks for me),
I'm spent from night after night of little sleep.
And I'm afraid today will echo the weekend.
If it does, how will I cope?
Oh Lord, help me!

Tuesday morning

Why did this insane catnapping and inconsolable
      crying
have to continue yesterday, Lord?
Why, why, why?
In one especially frightening moment last night,
our baby's shrieks were so loud and high-pitched and
      unrelenting
that we thought he was dying from crying.
I'm a wreck, Lord.
And the dog is a wreck;
the near-constant crying has upset him
to the point of incontinence.
Our marriage is a wreck too;
we began finger pointing yesterday,
blaming each other for our baby's fits,
and a bad fight erupted by nightfall.

My husband left the house in a huff but soon came
    back
with two beautiful roses for me,
and we apologized
and agreed that we're in an extraordinary situation
    here
that will pass one day.
It will pass, won't it, God?
This morning another day looms ahead of us,
and we need your help in keeping the peace
under our shaky roof.
Lord help us!

Wednesday evening

Yesterday and today were two more horrid days,
    Lord.
When will it ever end?
Will our baby ever take a nap of decent length?
Will he ever sleep for a humane stretch of time at
    night?
Will he ever stop crying?
When he screamed unceasingly today, God,
I felt like yelling, "Shut up!"
I feel ashamed of this anger I'm feeling

toward my tiny, defenseless baby today.
Please forgive me, God.
I know I would never intentionally hurt my baby
and I thank you, Lord, for the gifts of compassion and
    restraint.
Please help the hordes of parents in our world who
    feel
they can't bear another second of their babies' crying
    fits.
And please, Lord, help me to endure this long night
    ahead.

Thursday afternoon

Dear God, my baby hasn't napped all day.
Twelve hours and no sleep whatsoever.
Not one tiny break for me.
I've had little back-up help from my family
during this nightmarish week, Lord,
and no help at all from baby-sitters;
I don't dare leave this screaming machine
with a poor, unsuspecting sitter
for fear she'd never return to our house.
Oh Lord, when will *you* help me?

Friday afternoon

I slept a grand total of about twenty minutes last
      night, Lord.

My baby gets a gold star for the worst night on
      record.

I called the clinic this morning, choking on tears,

and insisted that a doctor or nurse see us today.

At the appointment this afternoon,

I was so weepy I could barely speak

but I managed to answer all of the nurse's questions

about our miserable week,

and an hour later she concluded, to my surprise,

"Your baby has colic."

She gave us some medicine to curb our baby's gas
      pains,

and revamped my dietary guidelines,

and reworked our breastfeeding schedule

to make breastfeeding easier on our baby's stomach.

Leaving the clinic, the day suddenly filled with
      sunshine, Lord,

and peace settled over our small family as we drove
      home.

Our little cherub seemed to sense that the nurse

had handed us hope for better days,
and he dropped into a deep sleep, right there in the
     car seat.

I'm so grateful for the explanation
we received at the clinic, Lord;
I never suspected our baby's behavior was colic.
Now we have hope for happier days.
But still, God, some trepidation remains—
I fear the trauma may continue.
If it does, Lord, please help us cope until this colic
     ends.

∾

Heaven-sent Baby Shower Presents

Thank you again, Lord, from the depths of my heart,
for protecting our baby and his small family two
    weeks ago,
the Sunday of his fifth week of life.
My husband filled the spare tire with air
at the gas station that Sunday,
and a few minutes later, as we drove through town,
that tire exploded in the trunk of the car.
The tire could have blown up
in my husband's face at the air pump,
hurting him terribly—or worse.
But you protected him, Lord,
and by shielding our baby's beloved daddy from
    harm,
you directly protected our baby.
Thank you, God!

It seems you've constantly blessed us
these two weeks since then, Lord—
a belated baby shower from heaven!
Much has improved under our roof
between week five and week seven postpartum;
our home's atmosphere and our outlook have
brightened remarkably.

Thank you, God,
for the fantastic baby present
we received on our baby's five-week birthday:
he slept a five-hour-long stretch in the night—his
        best ever!
Life again holds hope of becoming sane!
Thank you, God,
that the anti-gas drops the nurse gave us for our
baby's colic seem to have miraculously
taken the terrible edge off the crying fits;
at seven weeks of age, our baby is suddenly pacifiable
for long periods of time
simply by holding him closely on a grown-up's warm
        shoulder.
Thank you, God,
that now, in our baby's seventh week of life,

he's sleeping more soundly and in longer stretches by
     night
and in not–quite–so–brief catnaps by day.
Thank you, God,
for the relief that shared parenting can bring
and for the supplemental bottle my husband
has begun to feed the baby at night,
which gives me the respite I so desperately need
from round–the–clock breastfeeding.
Thank you, God,
that our baby is communicating with us
so beautifully now;
he coos delightfully when he's content
and whimpers heart-tuggingly when he's upset—
quiet little crying spells that are infinitely easier
on his parents' ears and nerves.
And he now laughs in his sleep—
a lovely sound that sends my heart into my throat
     with emotion.
Thank you, God,
that my baby smiled widely and directly at his
mommy this week—
a joy-filled first for me.
Thank you, God,

for all of these heaven-sent blessings
you've showered upon our small family
between week five and week seven postpartum.
Most of all, thank you, God,
for giving us this child.
He is simply the world's dearest, most adorable,
and darling baby.

Feeling His Pain

It's our sweet baby's eight-week birthday today, Lord,
and an unhappy birthday it's been.
He had his two-month checkup at the doctor's office
    this morning
and received three birthday presents he hated:
a stab with a long, sharp needle in one thigh,
another excruciating piercing in the other thigh,
and a dashed sense of trust in adults.
Our darling, unsuspecting baby was all-trusting and
    all-smiles
when we laid him on the table—
then his beloved parents just stood there and allowed
this horrible thing to happen to him.
He screamed and cried in pain during the shots
and for a long time afterward,
and I felt such anguish for him that I cried too.
I rocked him and rubbed his head and arms,

whispering "Oh honey" over and over.
My baby is a part of me, Lord.
I feel his pain.

Oh Lord God, help us!
Our baby awoke from a four-hour-long,
post-traumatic-doctor-visit nap,
and he has shrieked for a full half hour.
My husband and I are both terribly worried, Lord.
Is it lingering pain in his thighs from the needle pricks?
Is it a mild case of illness from the DPT immunization?
Or is our worst fear coming to pass?
We know there's a very, very remote chance that a baby
could be brain damaged from the DPT immunization.
We also know that an unusual high-pitched cry could
        indicate
a bad reaction to the vaccine.
Please comfort our baby, Lord,
and embrace him with your healing hands.

Lord, thank you for hearing my prayer.
Our baby's crying fit ceased and he fell asleep at last.
Now he's awake again and a changed child—
our amiable, smiling baby has reappeared.
Thank you, God, for this blessed restoration!

Spreading Sunshine

Now that our baby's colic is behind us,
a new baby is emerging before us, Lord.
"All I have to do is look at him
and he makes me smile," my husband says,
and the same is true for me.
We're getting the hugest kick
out of our baby now, God!
He grins these broad grins
and laughs this robust laughter,
spreading sunshine wherever he goes.
A neighbor visited us last night
and our baby flashed her a king-size grin.
We all laughed
and smiles spread throughout the room.
I'm thrilled to see my baby's personality budding
so soon in his young life.
Thank you, God, for this gladness, this delight!

Post-Baby Family Life

Fearing an Untimely Good-bye

In these first nine weeks of my new baby's life,
nightmarish images have darted through my mind, Lord,
arising out of my fear of Sudden Infant Death Syndrome.
If I lost my baby now, I don't know how I'd cope.
He'd be gone so soon, before we even got to know him,
before he'd taken his first step,
before he'd spoken his first word,
before he'd placed his first sweet kiss on his mommy's
    cheek.
My baby has, without question, given my life
more meaning than it's ever had before.
Losing our baby would leave such an enormous void in
    my life.
My pregnancy, the nursery preparations,
the hard weeks of colic,
and my dreams for our family's future,
all of this would seem pointless.

I fear my baby's physical death
would cause my spiritual death.
How would I cope, Lord?

If my baby died of SIDS or any other disorder, Lord,
I'm afraid, at some point, I'd be angry at you,
believing that you *could* have prevented it from happening.
Please, God, help me to comprehend your role in death,
especially in untimely deaths.
I have no doubt of your precious promise, Lord,
that if my baby died prematurely on earth,
he'd be alive and waiting for me in heaven.
Thank you, God, for the peace that comes from this
        promise.

I pray today, Lord, for all of the new parents in our world
whose lives have lost meaning
due to the untimely loss of their babies.
Please help these grieving parents
find ways to cope and carry on,
and offer them renewed hope for their families' futures.
Please comfort them with the conviction that one day
they'll have beautiful reunions with their babies in heaven.

Routines in Ruins

Our baby is nine weeks old now, Lord,
and something wondrous happened this week—
for several days in a row our little angel took longer
        naps,
not his usual disappointingly-short catnaps,
but true naps of decent length, two per day,
and at the same time each day.
Do you know what this means to me?
It means predictability.
Now I can plan my days
and actually hope to get some of my work done!

Our baby is ten weeks old now, Lord,
and I'm so upset I could cry.
So much for planning and predictability.
The longer naps didn't last
and he's back to catnapping.

For two months I've tried to protect him
from dreaded cold germs and flu bugs,
suspecting that the routines we've worked so hard to
     establish
would crumble in the face of a first illness.
And they have, Lord.
Just when we were all beginning
to sleep blissfully longer stretches at night—
four to five hours a stretch—
this cold brought on loud coughing, inconsolable crying,
and labored breathing.
And just when our breastfeeding routine had become
pleasant and predictable,
this cold brought on a feeding strike
because our baby is too stuffed-up to suckle.
I've had to pump my painfully engorged breasts night
     and day
and feed him the expressed milk with an eyedropper,
which is very tiring and time-consuming.
And just when our little cherub had begun
to play independently for longer periods—
meaning I could tackle chores and actually complete
     them—
this cold has made him terribly needy.

He wants to be held all the time
(when I try to put him down he wails pathetically)
so my arms, shoulders, and back ache
from lugging him around all day.
Other routines have, as expected,
toppled into ruins too, Lord.
I haven't had a second at my desk
and my work-related anxieties are skyrocketing.
I haven't been able to sleep, eat, or groom adequately.
I can barely get to the bathroom in time when I have
      to go.
What kind of life is this, God?
Please grant me strength and insight
to help me through this trying time.

Our dear baby has been sick all week, Lord,
suffering from too-little sleep
and struggling to breathe through his stuffed-up nose.
I've been miserable this week, too,
since his first cold has stolen
what precious little free time I have,
and I feel as if it's stolen my remaining bits of sanity.
I know this sounds selfish,
but time is so hard to find these days.

Our baby's discomfort should be my main concern
    this week,
not our daily routines.
Please, God, remind me of this.

I wish that now our post-baby family life
could settle into some kind of routine,
with some hope that it might stay that way.
Not knowing what to expect is very upsetting to me,
    Lord.
Our baby's future illnesses will likely have this same
    impact
and so will his many stages of development.
This makes me apprehensive about the future, Lord.
I can't count on much anymore.

Lord, please forgive me for viewing my baby's first cold
    so selfishly.
Please help him to recover soon.
Please help me to accept gracefully the reality
of our present life:
that sometimes our new routine will be no routine.

Thank you, Lord, for the constancy and dependability
of our love for our dear little one,
my husband's and my love for each other,
and your love for our family.

No Other Mother Knows

Never before in my life, Lord, have I felt as utterly alone
as I'm beginning to feel now in the fourth month
    postpartum.
It seems there's no one who fully understands
my troubles and stress
as a two-job mom who breastfeeds round-the-clock
and can't afford quite enough child care—
no one, not my husband, not my mother,
not my mother-in-law,
not my employers, not my colleagues,
not my childless friends, not even my friends who have
    children.
Some days, Lord, I feel as if I've sighed sunup to sunset
with weariness from explaining
why I can't have lunch,
why I'm too tired for a visit,
why I can't volunteer to serve on more committees,

why I don't have the time or energy
to celebrate a holiday weekend at the cabin.
It's so frustrating for me, Lord,
that many older mothers seem to have forgotten
how demanding it is to raise babies.
I'm trying to combine the job of raising a baby
with several major writing and editing projects at
    my desk,
and sometimes I feel resentful
because I have so little time
outside of work and baby care each day.
Please, Lord, help clear my heart of this resentment.

All new moms must feel lonely and misunderstood,
    Lord, just like I do.
Thank you for being there for me, God.
Thank you for your thorough understanding.
The affirmation I so desperately need comes from you
and makes me feel much less alone.
Please comfort me, Lord,
and help me to offer a consoling word
or lend a helping hand to other new mothers
    whenever possible.

Uproot the Bitter-fruit Tree, Lord

Among the many joy-bearing trees
in my inner orchard as a new mother,
a sour-fruit tree is also growing in my heart, Lord.
These bitter fruits are feelings of resentment and
      jealousy,
and I pray today for your help in uprooting the tree
that's bearing them.

I know it's my responsibility to care for my baby
and to remain dedicated to my career duties,
because these are the life choices I've made.
But I resent that I've received inadequate time,
      attention,
and assistance with my new baby
during these first difficult weeks, Lord.
Many days are still so hard,

especially since my baby remains a chronic catnapper,
which means too-brief breaks for me.
I imagined that people would line up outside our
    door
and beg to babysit
and clamor to help me out in a spectrum
of therapeutic ways.
But that fantasy is far from reality
and I feel isolated, neglected, needy, and angry.
My husband shook his head at me last night and said,
"You can't be angry with people for not meeting
    your needs,
when they have no idea what your needs are."
Now, I know this on an intellectual level, Lord,
but my emotions are another matter.
I feel people ought to *know*
without my having to tell them
that these have been the hardest weeks I've ever
    experienced
and that I need help.
But I guess this is unfair of me,
since most people aren't mind readers.
I'm aware that the books tell tired new moms to ask
    for help,

but I have a very hard time doing that, Lord,
since I've been fiercely independent forever
and feel awkward and uncomfortable asking for help.
I hate it!
Dear Lord, please teach me how to ask for help
when I need it and deserve it,
and please release me from this hurtful pride and anger.

Another bitter fruit growing in my inner orchard
is jealousy, Lord.
While I feel I'm not receiving enough help,
I see other new moms who are granted so much more
          than I've had.
One of my friends has family members who babysit
          every week,
and another has family members who babysit entire
          weekends.
I marvel at the way some of my friends can ask for help
without appearing to feel an ounce of guilt or
          reservation.
I wish I could be this assertive, but I'm not.
Please, Lord, teach me to be assertive
and release me from this hurtful jealousy.

Clashes in Wedlock

You know I've always had trouble, Lord,
feeling comfortable around people who are different
    than me—
not in skin color or religion, but in lifestyle—
such as people who wear bathrobes all day
and people who sleep until noon on weekends.
Even as a small girl, when I visited friends' homes
and saw their ways of life, sometimes I felt unsettled
and wanted to go home.
My difficulty accepting or appreciating differences in
    lifestyle
has taken on a profound meaning this year, Lord,
and I'm suddenly facing an all-new stranger
with a foreign lifestyle—
    my husband.

Dear Lord,
you know that my husband and I had our differences

in our life together pre-baby,
but they've sharpened in contrast since our baby's
     arrival,
and our list of differences has lengthened
during these first five months of new parenthood.
We differ in parenting styles:
I think the house should be quiet when the baby
     sleeps;
he thinks the baby should get used to some noise
at night and at naptime.
We differ in time-management choices:
I don't understand why he chooses to bake
a double batch of chocolate chip cookies
on a Saturday afternoon,
when there are so many chores to be done,
especially now, when the amount of time
for accomplishing necessary tasks is so limited.
Even the cores of our very personhood
seem to differ more radically now:
He's a night owl, I'm an early bird;
I can't stand clutter, he doesn't notice it;
I'm very organized, he's not;
I'm a work-before-play person, he prefers play
     before work;

I like things quiet, he was born loud.
I ask him to be quiet when the baby's sleeping
and he says he will,
then two minutes later he blows his nose like a
  foghorn
and clomps down the stairs in his big boots.
Our baby isn't the world's soundest sleeper, God,
and it appears as if my husband doesn't even *try*
to be quiet sometimes.
Dear God, I know 1 Corinthians 13
tells us that "love is not irritable,"
but that seems like a tall order in our present home
  life.
The combination of too little sleep and too much
  work
during these five months postpartum
has our irritability reaching volcanic states
and has us engaged in loud battles with locked horns.
Some days our differences seem to arise almost hourly
and lead to conflict at nearly every turn.
It's utterly tiresome.
Dear Lord, my husband and I desperately need
your guidance and spiritual gifts.
We are both concerned about the effect

our discord may have on our dear baby.
Please shower our union with the gifts of patience,
        kindness,
understanding, and acceptance.
Please help us to discover ways to resolve our
        differences
constructively rather than destructively.
Our little one is so pure and happy and in love with life,
and we fear our bickerings will darken his sunny outlook.
Please, God, help us remedy these trouble spots now
and renew us in true love.

Oh Lord,
my husband and I just had yet *another* difference of
        opinion,
and I don't care that I just slammed the bedroom door
and left him alone downstairs to tend to the crying baby
while I cry my own eyes out
up here on the bed.
When will the dissension ever end, God?
When, when, *when?*

Thank you, Lord, for a quick answer to that question.
I only had to wait five minutes for your answer.

My husband just came into the bedroom,
looked straight into my bloodshot eyes,
and said, "I love you."
In hearing those three little words,
my large load of anger and irritability melted away
and you answered my question, Lord:
dissension ends in love.
The differences may remain,
but the strife dissipates.
If I could ask for only one gift of the spirit this year
to help my small family
through these first troublesome months postpartum,
it would be love.
Please, Lord, bless this new mommy and this new
        daddy
with love in abundance.

&

Busy Baby, Busy Days

Dear God, calm the thunderclaps in my heart!
I turned my back just long enough to sort some dirty
    laundry,
then turned around—just in time—to find my baby
    hanging
halfway off the edge of my bed,
    head–first,
hovering high above the hardwood floor
and inching his way closer to calamity.
Falling off that tall bed onto that hard floor
could have seriously hurt my vulnerable baby.
I had set him in the center of my bed,
never suspecting his first inchworm locomotion
    would occur
this very afternoon.
Suddenly, in this third week of our baby's fifth month
    of life,

he can move in a way he's never been able to before.
Thank you, God, from the bottom of my pounding
      heart
for the vigilance of my baby's personal angel today.

New physical feats mean new and unexpected dangers
in ways I might not always anticipate, Lord.
As our baby swiftly approaches the half-year mark,
his rapid development is adding demands
to his mommy and daddy's surveillance duties.
His growth and development are quickly multiplying
the odds of baby-caused accidents occurring.
Please help us protect our baby from harming himself,
      Lord.

I fear more parent-caused accidents
may harm our baby now too, Lord,
since our household is suddenly busier than ever.
Just last Friday afternoon, my husband and I scrambled
      to leave
for a work-related meeting across town.
In the frantic chaos of packing the car,
we forgot to buckle our dear, irreplaceable baby
into his car seat.

After many miles of busy freeway driving, we arrived
only to discover our child's horrifying lack of
        protection.
Thank you, God, from the depths of my heart
for protecting our baby during that dangerous car
        ride,
and please continue to help us with the big job
of protecting our precious little one.

A Momentous First: Missed!

Thanksgiving Day morning

I'm sure you've heard my crying this holiday
        morning, Lord,
and you haven't heard the last of it.
Neither has my husband!
I went to bed early last night,
trusting my parenting partner would put the baby to
        bed later
with a nightcap of formula in a bottle.
My husband did that—and more—
but it's the "more" part that has me heartbroken.
This morning my dearly beloved reported the
        distressing news:
"I gave the little guy a bowl of rice cereal last night,
to see if he'd sleep better. He did well eating from a
        spoon."
That first spoonful of cereal last night
was the very first bite of solid food

in my baby's entire life,
and I missed it, Lord.
After nearly six months of exclusively breastfeeding,
when I've been his sole source of nourishment,
the start of solid foods means a giant step towards
        independence
for both my baby and me.
This is one of those things that only occurs once in a
        lifetime,
an act never to repeat itself.
Firsts only happen once, God,
and I missed this momentous one.
I'm feeling its loss like hunger pains in my stomach
        today.
Please, Lord, ease my sadness on this grey
Thanksgiving morning.

Thanksgiving Day evening

After lengthy and teary explanations on my part
        today, Lord,
my husband understands why this rice-cereal fiasco
        upset me so.
Now we're home again from our out-of-town
holiday day trip,

and before our baby retires for the night,
my husband has decided to whip up a batch of rice
        cereal
and recreate the momentous first solid-food feed,
        for my benefit.

Here goes, God...
I've got the bowl of warm mush in my hand
and our sweet babe is all set, strapped in his feeding
        seat,
blinking his huge baby blues at the white goo on the
        spoon
which I'm moving closer, closer to his perfect little lips
which he's opening wider, wider—
and in goes the mush!
and click goes the camera!
Our baby, who suddenly appears so big and grown-up,
gums that mush in the cutest way
then swallows his very first introductory bite . . .
and whines for more. I can't believe this—
he's begging for more, Lord!
And he grabs the spoon out of my hand and tries to
        feed himself.
I'm totally amazed!

He gobbles up bite after bite
and his face, ears, head, and pajamas are covered with
        cereal.
Just listen to those little lips lick and smack.
This is a complete marvel, Lord!

Dear God, now I can say "Happy Thanksgiving" and
        really mean it.
Thank you that this reenacted event felt to me
like the very first official feed of my baby's life.
Thank you for triumphant milestones, for jubilant firsts.
Thank you for my dear husband who, I know, always
        does his best.
Thank you for all times when spouses
come to understand each other,
when heartwounds are healed and broken moments are
        rebuilt.
Thank you that my anger and sadness dissolved away
        today
like powdered cereal in milk.
Thank you, dear Lord, for our good fortune
in having food on our table this Thanksgiving Day,
with which to feed our hungry little one.

෫

Half Birthday, Wholly Thankful

Our new family celebrated our first Thanksgiving
    together
two weeks ago, Lord,
and today we're celebrating another festive occasion—
our baby's half birthday!
We took a half-birthday photo of the little birthday
    star,
perched beside a half-cupcake topped with half of a
    candle.
I have so much gratitude in my heart, God,
at the halfway mark of my baby's first year on earth.

Thank you, Lord, that the peak period
when Sudden Infant Death Syndrome is most likely
    to strike is now over;

I feel immeasurably blessed that my baby and our
family
have been spared this nightmare.
Thank you that our baby is sleeping through the
night at last
and for the vast relief this brings to our family life.
Thank you that our baby plays more independently
now,
which gives his parents much-needed reprieves.
Thank you that our daily baby-care routines
have become more established,
which makes everything run more smoothly in our
home.
Thank you that our baby's second cold,
which he caught last week,
was infinitely easier than his first.
Thank you that lately we seem to witness our
curious,
ambitious baby perform a new feat almost daily.
Just since Thanksgiving he's learned
to clasp his hands together like a choirboy,
to roll from his back onto his tummy,
to blow bubbles with his food and drool,
and to drink from an infant cup,

insisting on holding the cup all by himself.
Thank you too, Lord, that with each new sunrise,
our baby's smile grows sweeter,
his sense of humor grows more ticklish,
he becomes more spellbindingly fun
and more kissably, huggably, and irresistibly cute.
Do all moms feel this way when their babies turn six
        months old?
If they do, you've blessed them richly, Lord.
Most of all, Lord, thank you
that my love for my baby
has now become reciprocal.
This precious little person swept me off my feet
the moment I first spied him at his birth.
Now I see he's beginning to fall in love with me too.
I see his recognition solidifying of who I am
and what I represent in his life.
He caresses my arm and chest slowly and gently
as he nurses at my breast;
he wraps his arms around my neck and clings on
        indivisibly,
burying his face in my shoulder and hair;
and he seems now to adore sharing these joyful
moments with me

just as much as I cherish spending them with him.
Every day, my husband and I stand awestruck in
    observing
this amazing little human we created together.
I feel so fortunate to be his mother.
Thank you, Lord, for bringing this blessed child into
    our lives.

Center of My Universe

The newest member of our small family
has become a supernova at the center of my universe,
　　Lord—
he's brought so much light to my life!
But lately I've begun to wonder:
is something wrong with having a diaper–clad
　　supernova
at the core of my world?
I do adore this child, Lord,
and he becomes more adorable with each new day.
The more charming our baby becomes, though,
the more my adoration of him seems to border on
　　worship.
I've secretly begun to worry, Lord,
that our baby might be an idol in my life,
my little golden calf in diapers.
In our early years of marriage,

my husband became the nucleus of my life;
my world revolved around him,
and now I'm afraid I'm repeating the same mistake
    with our baby.
Please remind me who the true center
of my universe is, Lord:
    you.
Only then will I know
real happiness and fulfillment.

New Challenges

Yet a Freshman Mother

It's been seven months since my baby's birth
and I feel like I'm facing the complete unknown
all over again, Lord.
My baby's suddenly entering all-new developmental
      phases,
which means once again I have to try to comprehend
a barrage of new child-care information.
I feel nearly as ignorant and unqualified
as I did on day one postpartum
when I had so many questions.
Once more, I feel like a floundering freshman
attending Baby Care University.
I'm facing new questions
about sleep patterns, baby equipment, day-care centers,
      weaning,
childproofing, socializing, discipline, and starting solids.
I feel tired and weary even before I begin,

and I'm slow and reluctant to begin the more
challenging tasks—
such as looking for a day-care situation
that would be acceptable to me.
Dear God, please clear my confusion and renew my
    confidence
as I search for these answers
and grant me the strength necessary to face these new
    challenges
as caretaker of this maturing child.

I'm facing another new challenge now too, Lord:
a test of my patience.
When my baby pulls his socks off and chomps on them,
when he throws his toys all around the house,
when he blows bubbles with his food,
showering me with mashed peas and carrots,
when he's so distracted during a breastfeeding session
that he hangs upside-down off my lap
and wiggles and wrestles and does anything but nurse,
when he flails around on the changing table,
making clothing and diaper changes as difficult
as trying to dress a wild boar,
when he rolls over onto his tummy on the playmat

and gets stranded like a turtle in his inability to roll back
and whines and cries until I flip him over again,
my tolerance is tested to the extreme
and my sighs ascend to record-high decibel levels.
Dear Lord, please grant me the patience
and the sense of humor I need
to endure these new developmental phases with grace.

Your blessings of patience, confidence, and courage,
    Lord,
will help me to undertake my course work
at this Baby Care University with greater success.
Maybe someday I'll graduate with a major in
    motherhood
but I'm afraid I won't receive my diploma for years.
Please, Lord, as my mommy-in-the-making education
    continues,
help me to relax and accept the fact
that I don't have all the correct answers, and never will.
Please help me to enjoy the process of learning
and to relish the time spent with my challenging
yet absolutely charming little baby.

The Load of Adulthood

Some days, as I lay our little angel down for a nap,
     Lord,
and pull his cozy blanket up to his chin
and watch him drift off to visit Mr. Sandman,
I long to be in my slumbering infant's place.
My baby has no demands on his days
other than to eat, sleep, play, giggle,
and watch the world go by.
I'm feeling the load of adulthood, Lord,
and I realize how heavily the responsibilities
of chores, work, and child-care duties
have weighed on my shoulders
since my baby's birth nearly eight months ago.
If only I could shed the weight whenever I felt
     overburdened,
to give my soul, spirit, muscles, and mind
a chance to recuperate,

then all would be well.
But it seems that the load of adulthood
is permanently strapped to my back now.
I know my responsibilities for my child will continue
into his own adulthood.
And there's no altering the permanence
of my other responsibilities in life.
I've become more aware these past eight months
of the young, childless couple that lives next door,
        Lord.
I observe their lifestyle wistfully from across the fence,
noticing that they go out many evenings—
probably to movies, plays, parties, museums, restaurants.
I notice their late-morning breakfasts on their deck
when they read, it seems, the *complete* newspaper.
Of course they have chores to do and must go to
        their jobs,
but they don't have a baby,
and from across the fence, their load appears
        featherweight
in comparison to mine.
I feel like a pack animal lately, Lord,
saddled with a massive load of adult duties
and grown-up concerns.

This is the first time I've talked to you in several days,
    Lord.
Some days I'm so busy and tired
that I don't take even a minute to talk with you.
I know my load lightens and my outlook brightens
when I share my problems with you in prayer.
Thank you, Lord, for listening to my prayers
and for your answers.

Longer Trips to Dreamland

Dear Lord, I am immensely grateful
for the heaven-sent gift I received this eighth month
    postpartum.
After all of these months of chronic catnapping,
fifteen minutes here, twenty minutes there—
distressingly short bits of fitful sleep—
our baby has finally begun to take daily naps of decent
    length,
an hour or more each, two per day, and at predictable
    times.
To me, Lord, the most precious commodity in the
    world
isn't money, it isn't diamonds, it's time.
My baby's longer trips to dreamland
mean more precious spare time for his mommy.
This week I actually tackled projects from start to finish
and crossed items off my lengthy list of things to do.

And this afternoon I actually sat on my bed,
sipped a cup of coffee,
curled up my tired legs,
and read a book—for a *whole hour* while the baby
    napped!
There aren't words to express the magnitude of my
    gratitude
for these daily reprieves, Lord.
Thank you, God, for the priceless gift
of a baby's long, sound nap.

Unblemished Babies

Our friends just had a baby girl, Lord,
and she's not even a week old, yet her parents report
that she's already sleeping long, sound stretches at
    night,
she's already breastfeeding beautifully,
and every member of her new small family
is in fine, delightful shape.
When I hear of babies who sleep well from the
    outset,
or other "perfect baby" stories,
I can't help but feel envious as I recall
our own baby's fitful nights of sleep
during his early months of colic
and his seven-plus months of frustratingly short
    catnaps.
These memories are now, in the ninth month
    postpartum,

still fresh in my mind and probably always will be.
Dear God, please help me to be generous in spirit
and deliver me from jealousy
when I hear tales about other babies.

If I were to be honest with you, Lord, and honest
        with myself,
I'd admit that the "perfect baby" is a myth.
I told my mother last night
how disheartening it is to hear perfect-baby stories,
and she replied, "But *you* have a perfect baby."
I reminded her of his colic and catnaps,
to which she said firmly, "But *now* he's perfect."
It's true, Lord,
our friends and even total strangers echo my mother's
        sentiment:
"What a charming, delightful, beautiful, perfect baby
you have" tends to be the refrain.
In the second half of our baby's first year of life,
he's become exceedingly wonderful,
and I'm pretty quick to proclaim this to the entire
        universe.
So perhaps I've been telling some of my own
perfect-baby stories without realizing it.

And I suppose these stories may have had the same
     affect
on some new mothers as similar stories have effected me.

Please, Lord,
help me to hold back from comparing my baby to others
or other babies to mine
if it's going to hurt me
or hurt other moms
or hurt the children themselves.
I hope I haven't already ensnared another mom
in the comparison trap, Lord,
and please heal her hurt feelings if I have.
Help me to see my verbal error, if I've already made one,
and help me to avoid repeating the same mistake in the
     future.
And please, Lord, help me to erase the idea of the
     "perfect baby"
entirely from my mind.

A Wellspring of Joy

It seems that every day now, God,
this nine-month-old charmer
brings a spectrum of joyful emotions to my world!

Our baby's begun to pull his big toe up to his mouth
        and suck on it,
his eyes twinkling in amusement—
a new trick that makes his daddy and me laugh.
Thank you, God, for this silliness!

Our baby had the first swing ride of his life
at the playground this week
and he loved every second of it,
throwing back his head and squealing with glee
at every push of the swing.
Thank you, God, for this exhilaration!

Our baby received a white plush bunny from his
    grandma
on Easter Sunday two weeks ago,
and he still giggles every time he sees it
and squishes the fuzzy bunny into his face.
Thank you, God, for this merriment!

Our baby has suddenly taken an intense interest in
    picture books
and it's adorable when he tries to pick the objects
off the page with his index finger
and when he gazes upon the pages of *upside-down* books,
studying them for the longest stretches of time.
Thank you, God, for this endearment!

Our baby and I sometimes waltz
to a beautiful classical piece on Public Radio
and in a gentle embrace with him placed on my hip,
I see him smile as we slowly circle the room
and my heart dances too.
Thank you, God, for this intimacy!

Our baby lay on the changing table today,
remaining still the entire time I changed him.

With his head turned to the side
and his slowly blinking eyes gazing out the window,
his hands remained clasped angelically together
and I was convinced that all this little cherub lacked
was a set of wings.
Thank you, God, for this winsomeness!

Our baby sometimes drifts off
as I rock him briefly before his nap
and I'm certain that nothing in the world is sweeter
than the feeling of this baby's little nose and moist
    mouth
nuzzled against my neck as he falls asleep in my arms.
Thank you, God, for this tenderness!

Our baby and his daddy giggled and rolled around
on the living room floor last night
and afterwards, his daddy walked into the kitchen
    and sighed.
"Why the sigh?" I asked.
"He's just so *cute*," my husband replied,
beside himself with admiration.
Thank you, God, that this baby is bringing such delight
to his daddy's world too!

This little one has become a wellspring of joy in our
       lives,
which now is flowing more than ever before, Lord.
Thank you for every one of these cherished
       moments.

Irretrievable Babyhood

Our baby turned nine months old this week, Lord,
and I noticed that our dog looked *small*
sitting beside our growing boy!
I can hardly believe this big baby
with his fat tummy, hearty laugh, and gap-tooth grin
who sits without support now
and who crawls like a speed-racing centipede
was inside me and only the size of a peach
just one year ago.
At nine months, my baby has reached the three-
 quarter mark;
he's entering the twilight of his first year of life,
and it's a bittersweet time for me, Lord.
Of course it's thrilling to watch him grow up,
but he'll never be this little again,
and I'll miss his littleness when it's gone.
I felt the first stirrings of this sadness

in his second month of life
when I packed away his tiniest clothes
that he'd already outgrown.
I felt this pang of loss again in the fourth month
when we moved him from his bassinet in our bedroom
into the crib in the nursery
where he began to spend nights and naptimes all by
    himself.
I feel panicky sometimes, Lord,
when I suspect my baby's irretrievable babyhood
is slipping away too soon
and that it will leave me
before I'm ready to bid it good-bye.

I often feel the need, Lord, to hold onto this fleeting
    time.
I'm thankful for photographs, videotapes, and journals
that help preserve these precious moments.
I'm also reassured in knowing that my baby
still has a lot of "little" years left.
Thank you Lord,
that though our baby can appear so grown-up one
    minute,
when he's crawling in the living room at full speed,

the next minute he can look tiny again,
when he's curled up on his daddy's chest.
Remind me, Lord, to relish my baby's littleness
every moment that I'm able while it lasts.
And help me to find comfort in the truth
that although one day I'll no longer have my tiny
    baby
to hold in my arms,
I will always have his babyhood memories
to hold in my heart.

Angels to
My Aid

A Houseful of Germs

I ache in every single bodily muscle this morning, Lord.
I'm running a temperature of 102° Fahrenheit,
and my head feels like somebody stomped on it.
I guess this means I'll take a sick day, God,
my first official sick day since my baby's birth ten
     months ago.
I won't do laundry or dishes.
I won't work at my desk while the baby naps.
I won't run errands or take the baby to the park.
This day has but one purpose: convalescence.
I'll lie down when my little one naps today,
and, baby willing, I'll be granted an easy day of child
     care too.

I tried to give myself a sick day, Lord,
but my baby wouldn't cooperate.
He's caught this nasty virus also

and in his misery has cried most of the day
and refused to be put down.
My already aching muscles now ache doubly
after lugging this huge ten-month-old child around for
      hours.
With my baby hanging heavily on one arm,
I performed Olympian maneuvers with the other:
sponging up the breakfast he vomited all over the
      nursery floor;
wiping up the pool of pink liquid antibiotic
that he spilled all over the kitchen floor;
mopping up the monstrous b.m. mess that oozed out of
his diaper and up his back and down his legs
and all over his clothes and the changing table too,
when I just couldn't understand why this huge mess had
      to happen
today of all days!
Throughout this day, Lord, my head has pounded,
the swollen glands in my throat have made every
      swallow hurt,
I've felt faint and feverish,
and every minute I've longed to lie down,
but my baby wouldn't let me—except when he napped,
a break that felt much too brief to me today.

O Lord, thank you for the beautiful sound I just heard:
my husband's car pulling in the driveway.
My heart swells with emotion just seeing him walk in
     the door.
I peel the baby off me and hand him over,
then shed several tears on my husband's shoulder,
then drag myself upstairs and crawl into bed.
I wasn't granted a sick day today, God,
but I have the evening off,
and for that I am eternally grateful.

I realize babysitters will be scarce
during our family's illnesses, Lord,
since inviting people to visit a houseful of germs
     is inappropriate.
So thank you, Lord, for my good fortune
in having a helpful husband in my life.
Thank you for all individuals who provide relief
to overburdened moms in times of trouble and undue
     stress.
Please, Lord, send aid—in any form you see fit—
to all those mothers in our world
who don't have even one person to assist them in
     difficult times.

Saying No

It's six o'clock p.m., Lord, time for the nightly news,
and my own report of this day on the home front isn't
        pretty.
Our baby's still sick with this terrible virus,
the bug is lingering in my system too,
plus we're all exhausted from several consecutive nights
of illness-induced poor sleep.
In my baby's discomfort today he didn't nap for a
        minute,
he didn't allow me even the tiniest little break,
so of course I accomplished nothing at my desk.
And I feel weak too—not just from the virus—
but from hunger, since I barely had time to eat all day.
I also feel as greasy as this hamburger
that I'm trying to fry on the stove here,
since I wasn't granted a moment for a shower since
        sun-up.

What a day, Lord. What a life!
And our evening holds little promise of improvement,
since my dear babe is refusing to eat his dinner,
and just threw his peas and pasta onto the floor,
and is screeching to be released from his high-chair.
I trust the moment I set him down
he'll latch onto my legs and whine and cry
and refuse to allow his starving mother
the chance to finish making her dinner.
And there goes the phone.
Now what, Lord?
My husband is already late in coming home;
if that's him calling to say he's going to be even later,
I'm going to scream.
Lord, please help me not to scream.
Please help me to control this tongue of mine.

Right in the middle of my dinnertime mayhem,
a woman from church introduced herself over the
        telephone
and said, "We want you to be on our refugee
        committee."
Exasperated, I felt like asking her,
"Do you realize who you're calling?

Did *you* serve on committees when your children
were tiny babies?
Did *you* also work at a demanding job that required
almost every one of your spare minutes
outside of chores and baby care?"
Thank you for helping me hold my tongue, Lord.
I simply said, "No. I can't now because of work and
     the baby.
But I would like to help in the future,
when demands on my time ease."

I'm worn out, Lord.
I'm wrung out.
Yet part of me wishes I could have said yes
to the woman at church.
Could I, somehow, make time to serve on that
     committee?
Do you want me to?
I feel tremendously guilty saying no, Lord.

There's no denying it,
this is a difficult time in my life.
I want to help the needy, Lord, but it seems an
     impossibility

when I feel so needy myself.
I wouldn't have much to offer that committee or
those refugees
with the minuscule time and energy
left in my depleted reserves.
Please renew my strength, Lord,
so that I may resume helping others.
And please show me how I can help.

One Month Later

Today as I picked a few dandelions in the yard, Lord,
a little Chinese girl stepped inside our fenced-in yard
and said to me, "My mother's really sad.
I'd bring my baby brother back from the dead if I
could.
But I can't. And there's nothing I can do
to make my mother happy."
I dropped my gardening gloves at once
and followed that little girl home.
There I found a very depressed woman,
in deep mourning over the death of her baby boy—
lost to a terminal illness at three months of age.
In broken English, this woman—
who emigrated from China four years ago—

recounted to me the story
of her baby's gradual and painful death,
confided in me her regrets over the time spent with
      her baby,
and shared with me the worst part of losing her child—
knowing how terribly he suffered during his short stay
      on earth.
For more than an hour, Lord,
this bereaved woman and I cried together
and I held her hand and listened,
and I tried to affirm her feelings
and acknowledge the tremendous care and love
that she had given her dying baby.
"I wish I could believe in God and heaven," she said,
"so I could know my baby is in heaven.
But because of the way I was raised in China, I cannot
      believe."
In a voice choked with emotion,
I shared my firm conviction with her:
"Take it from me.
Your baby is alive and well this very minute
and is in the safest care in heaven.
He has twenty nurses tending to him but he doesn't
      need them,

because he's in perfect health and is perfectly happy.
I have no doubt in my mind about this."
The woman smiled for the first time during our visit
and thanked me as we hugged each other good-bye.

A month ago I had to say no
to serving on that refugee committee, Lord,
but today you showed me how I could help an
immigrant family
in my own limited way.
Please, Lord, continue to show me
how I may be of service to people in need.

❧

Our Dear Child, Already Ruined

Dear Lord,
our ten-month-old little one
started a new habit this week that really has me
worried.
Every day now, all day long it seems,
our baby grinds his four front teeth together—
his two upper and two lower.
I'm afraid my husband's and my frantic lifestyle
and occasional upsets at home
have stressed our baby
and that he's grinding his teeth in nervousness.
I feel just awful, Lord.
I fear we've ruined our child already
and he's not even a year old!
Please show me quickly, God,
if there's anything at all I can do.

I took our sweet baby
with me to my writers' group this afternoon, Lord,
and he demonstrated his new teeth-grinding habit
to my colleagues.
I shared my worries with my writer friends—
my fears that our baby is a bundle of nerves already
and that it's all my fault.
One of my colleagues, an older mom, laughed and said,
"You're so funny!
He's rubbing his teeth together because it feels good,
not because of stress.
The rubbing relieves his teething pain."
"Oh," I replied with a smile.
What a great sense of relief, God!

I'm so thankful, Lord,
for those honey-laden, healing words that my colleague
        spoke
and for the relief they brought me today.
It's so good to have wise moms in my midst
who help put my fears, worries and self-blame to rest.
I'm very grateful, God,
for their knowledge, experience, and helpful insights.

❧

Visit from an Angel

Since our little one began to crawl, Lord,
I've feared that if he ever managed to maneuver his way
past the safety gate barring him from our family room,
he'd find himself crawling toward a nightmare:
the steep basement stairs that lead to the cement floor
    below.
A renovation project this spring
has left our basement entrance exposed, with no barrier.
It will be a couple of weeks
before the construction project is completed,
but our curious eleven-and-a-half-month-old crawler
let me know today, Lord, in no uncertain terms,
that completing the project quickly is a must.

After lunch today, I ran upstairs for a minute
to grab a change of clothes for the baby,
trusting he'd be fine by himself

for a brief moment on the main floor.
But soon after heading upstairs,
I realized that playtime downstairs
had become ominously quiet.
Sensing something was wrong, I dashed down the
          steps.
I ran through the living room—no baby,
through the dining room—no baby,
and into the kitchen—still, no baby.
O Lord, I hadn't latched that safety gate!
I leaped into the family room and saw my baby
perched at the top of the steep basement steps,
staring transfixed at the cement floor below.

The second I spied my baby hovering over that
          disaster trap,
a strange, matter-of-fact feeling came over me,
          Lord,
and I felt no panic.
Slowly, I walked over to him
and calmly picked him up.
At that moment,
I knew that my baby would *never* have fallen down
          those stairs,

because I truly believe that you've heard my fervent
      prayers
and that you sent your angels to my aid today.

Every minute of every day, Lord,
I assume responsibility for my baby's safety.
But there will be times, like today, when I'll slip up.
I realize now and wholeheartedly believe that my baby
wasn't staring transfixed at the basement floor today,
but rather at a beautiful angel
who wasn't about to let that baby tumble down those
      stairs.
I believe the shimmering image of that heavenly being
held my baby spellbound
until I arrived to gather him safely into my own arms.
Thank you for always being there for me, God,
in my demanding role as mother,
especially on days like today
when I need you the most.

Sunnier Days

I can hardly believe, Lord, that one week from today
our baby will turn *one year old!*
This gorgeous spring morning, I took the soon-to-be
    birthday boy
for a ride in his stroller and told him as we raced
    along,
"A year ago exactly I was bigger than a barn
and could hardly walk.
I was moving really slow with you in my tummy.
But look at us now!
I'm small again and you're so big.
And I'm light on my feet again too."
My baby laughed and swung his suntanned bare feet
and pointed at the robins and squirrels,
and I thought, We've both come a long way in one
    year's time!
Thank you, Lord, for change.

Thank you for brighter days which follow the dark ones.
Now, as a nearly one-year-old mommy,
I see that motherhood does get easier,
and I believe that babies do become more manageable.
In my troubled early months of new mommyhood,
I had a hard time imagining that our home life
would ever improve,
though experienced mothers tried to assure me it
    would.
The trials seemed never-ending then, Lord.
In the midst of our baby's colicky fits,
I never imagined that one day he'd become
the sweet-tempered charmer with the ready smile he is
    today.
And if someone had told me six months ago
that silliness, playfulness, and laughter would return
to my marital relationship, I would've replied,
    "I doubt it,"
but we're actually seeing a resurrection of levity, Lord!
Our home life has grown sunnier in *many* ways,
and I'm very grateful.

Still, Lord, some of our days can seem very dark
    even now,

and I lose hope that better days will follow the bleak
　　　ones
when my husband and I aren't communicating well;
when days are so busy from start to finish
that we barely have time to breathe;
when our sleep at night is interrupted yet again
by our baby who's in teething pain
and I wonder if I'll *ever* again in my life feel fully rested.
During times when parenting or our marital
　　　communication
becomes particularly troubled, Lord,
please renew my hope that happier days lie ahead
and that our small family's home life will continue to
　　　brighten.

Life is getting easier, Lord.
I'm crying "O God, help me!" far less often now
than I did in those earliest months postpartum.
But please, Lord, though my needs may be fewer now,
remind me to continue to call on you daily for guidance
and for your gifts of love, forgiveness, patience, and
　　　kindness,
which our family will always need.

❧

A New Means of Locomotion

Wednesday Night

Dear God, how more exciting could a birthday
    week get?
Our baby's first birthday is the day after tomorrow
and my husband and I sat in the living room tonight,
finalizing plans for the birthday party,
when our little one pulled himself to standing,
holding onto the couch,
then suddenly pushed away
and took one—two—three steps across the living
    room rug!
My husband and I gasped in awe
and laughed in delight
and I shouted, "Sweetheart, you're *walking*."
We just witnessed the very first steps of our child's
    life, Lord!

Thursday Night

Our baby set out on more expeditions today, Lord,
putting his new skills as a pedestrian to the test
and traveling even farther than yesterday—
as many as ten steps in a single outing.
He tottered through the dining room on tiptoe,
his fists clenched tightly and held high in the air for
     balance,
and managed nearly a dozen steps before teetering
and falling backward onto his behind.
"That's fantastic!" his daddy and I exclaimed in near
     disbelief
and applauded wildly every time he toddled across
     the room.
Equally excited, our baby squealed and laughed and
     clapped
during his travels today,
obviously thrilled by his new means of locomotion.

My husband and I are astonished
at this miracle unfolding before us, Lord.
This year we've seen a tiny, immobile, helpless baby
begin to creep,
then crawl,

then pull up,
then stand,
then take a first step,
and suddenly—walk!
It's breathtaking, Lord!
Thank you, God, for offering us such joy
as we witness the developmental feats
of our little wonder.

Happy Birthday!

Our dear little one
is one whole year old, Lord!
Never before could I understand parents
who invited everyone on the planet, it seemed,
to their children's first birthday parties,
but now I understand—
it's a tremendous cause for celebration!
Our baby has survived crib death
and we've all survived a monumental hurdle—
his first year of life.
Forty people came to our baby's party today, Lord,
and the huge bash launched him spectacularly into
    toddlerhood.
Thank you for our growing family's
innumerable reasons to celebrate today.

Thank you, Lord, for bringing into my life
the cutest creature that ever crawled the face of the
      earth.
Thank you for the affirmation I receive every single day
when my baby smiles his open smile
and laughs his deep hearty laugh
and throws his arms up in excitement—
when his happiness tells me that I'm being the best
      mommy
I can possibly be.
Thank you that my baby is now saying "Mama"—
two sweeter syllables do not exist in our world.
Thank you for every tender moment when my baby
      and I
cuddle and rock and laugh and play and sing and dance
      together.
Thank you that still, a year after my baby's birth,
when he lies by my side
and I stroke his smooth head and his perfect tiny ears,
I am beside myself with awe over this little breathing
      miracle.
Thank you, God, for the gift of life,
for our baby's life.

He seems so happy to be here.
He seems so glad he was born.
And his daddy's and my joy over his life
is absolutely boundless.

To top off the birthday celebration this evening,
we drove down to the lake, Lord,
and we walked along the beach,
and our baby saw his first ducks and paddle boats
and a shimmering rainbow right over the middle of
        the lake.
That rainbow was a glorious ornament
on our baby's first-birthday cake, Lord,
and I thank you for this gift.
My baby's first year of life has simultaneously been
the most pain-filled year
and the most joy-filled year
I've ever known.
Seeing that rainbow over the lake this evening was a
        fitting end,
a sign of promise that the worst of the storm is
        behind us
and a clear message from above
that our family remains in your care—

just as you've cared so lovingly for us
throughout our child's first year.
Thank you, Lord, for blessing us so richly
with this dear baby.

Safeguard Our Beloved Child

Simply Because a Mother Asks

⁓

July 3

I've decided it's time to wean
our nearly thirteen-month-old cherub from the breast,
	Lord.
Ever since his sixth month of life,
I've hoped he would take the lead and self-wean,
but he's clearly fond of breastfeeding
and has shown no signs of *ever* wanting to stop.
Ending this cozy relationship
and beautiful aspect of my baby's babyhood
fills me with sorrow
and a profound sense of loss, Lord.
But I feel even more worried than sad—
worried about any unhappiness weaning may bring to
	my baby.
The books tell me that babies receive the most comfort
from their early-morning and bedtime breastfeedings

and when these "comfort feeds" are denied,
babies often throw tantrums
and their routines are thrown into disorder.
I plan to drop the early-morning feed tomorrow,
then drop the bedtime feed a week later.
I'm expecting a difficult time,
with lots of inconsolable crying coming from the
    crib.
Dear Lord, please ease the predawn trauma
in our nursery tomorrow.
Please lessen our little one's sense of loss.

July 4, Independence Day

Your answer to prayer this Fourth of July morning
is as startling and awe-inspiring as a burst of fireworks,
    Lord!
When the baby woke up crying at 5:15 a.m.,
I stayed quietly out of sight.
My husband changed the baby's diaper,
offered him milk from a cup (which he didn't drink),
rocked and hugged him for several minutes,
then returned him to his crib.
Our little angel uttered one little whimper,
then fell back to sleep

and slept soundly until 7:30 a.m.
No tantrum.
No notable distress.
He fell back to sleep so peacefully
that both of us were astounded.
I firmly believe, Lord,
that this peaceful scene today was your design
and that you helped comfort our baby—
simply because a mother asked.

Weaning my baby from the breast is very sad for me,
    God.
But my child is becoming more independent of his
    mommy
and this is also liberating for me.
Thank you, dear Lord, on this Independence Day,
for this newfound sense of maternal liberation.

One Week Later
Last night, my baby experienced
the last breastfeed of his life, Lord,
but he didn't know it at the time.
I knew it though,
and I cried.

When my baby's bedtime arrives this evening,
he'll discover that his breastfeeding relationship
with his mommy has ended.
Dear Lord, please lessen my little one's feeling of loss
at his bedtime tonight,
and tomorrow night as well,
and please continue to do so
until breastfeeding becomes nothing more
than a vague and pleasant memory for him.

Baby's Bedtime

Oh thank you, God!
My husband gave our baby his bath,
offered him milk from a cup (which he drank),
then paced the nursery for a few minutes
with the baby wrapped in his favorite blanket,
and our little one fell sound asleep in his daddy's
      arms.
My breastfeeding relationship with my baby is over,
      Lord.
Thank you for comforting both my baby and me
as we say good-bye to this tender gift we shared.

You know how I fretted about my baby's well-being
during weaning, Lord!
May this experience always serve as a reminder to me,
in all my future years as a worrisome mother,
that freedom from anxiety over my child's well-being
is mine for the asking,
the moment I turn my troubles over to you.
I study the lovely face of my baby, Lord,
and I believe with conviction
that this is a child who will forever
remain in your care—
simply because a mother asks.

Social Trials

A hurricane of social blows struck
our sweet thirteen-month-old this weekend, Lord.
On Saturday, at a gathering of friends,
an older boy intentionally bulldozed our baby out of
      his way.
Our baby toppled over
and he cried.
We visited friends on Sunday
and two toddlers cornered our baby in the kitchen
      nook.
Our baby felt trapped and alarmed,
and he cried.
On Monday morning, an older playmate
repeatedly grabbed our baby's toys out of his hands.
Our baby felt bewildered and angry,
and he cried.
The painful process of socialization has begun, Lord.

Our child is swiftly discovering
that the world is a nasty place sometimes.
When I see my child harmed, Lord,
my own heart needs bandaging.
After witnessing the older boy bulldoze
our unsuspecting baby
out of his way,
my husband said, "I feel so bad for him.
It breaks my heart."
I want to leap in to rescue my little one
when he's harassed by a playmate, Lord.
But I know that eventually he'll have to learn to
     conquer
these social trials on his own,
since I won't always be able to be there
to serve as his defender.
During these times, God, please safeguard our beloved
     child.

The Following Weekend

O Lord, my little beauty
acted like a complete beast
at his playmate's house this morning!
I've never seen our dear baby act this aggressive before.

In a fit of jealousy
over the attention I paid to his playmate today,
my baby hit his little friend
and pulled his hair
and pinched his cheek in such a tight vice-grip
that I couldn't pry his fingers away in time
and his sharp nails cut through his poor
     playmate's skin
and drew blood.
I feel just terrible!
Suddenly and unexpectedly
we're seeing so soon in our baby's young life
his aggressive side.
It's frightening for me
and I'm sure it's frightening for him too.
Please, Lord, guide my child's hands and his heart
all the days of his life
so that the loving side of his nature
reigns supreme.

Home Improvements

My husband and I had a bad argument last night, Lord,
in front of our baby
and this morning we still fumed
and flung several hostile words at each other,
which our baby heard and witnessed.
Our little one spent the morning at his day-care center
and when I picked him up, his teacher reported
that our normally gregarious, sunny-natured child
was not at all himself today.
"He seemed so *sad*,"
the teacher told me with a look of concern.
"He wouldn't play with the other children.
When we all went outside to play,
his lip quivered and instead of playing with the others,
he crawled onto my lap
and fell asleep in my arms.
He just seemed very *sad* today."

I feel wretched, God.
My heart is in shreds
because our precious child saw his mommy and
    daddy
so mad at each other
and this caused him so much sadness today.

Dear Lord,
help my husband and me remember to disagree
    respectfully
and work toward resolutions peacefully
when our conflicts begin to become hurtful and
    volatile.
Since my baby's birth fifteen months ago,
I've been deluding myself in believing that destructive
    fighting
wouldn't affect our child adversely if he witnessed it.
But I've seen today, too clearly, that it does.
If my husband and I had reconciled
before our child left for school this morning—
making sure he'd witnessed us kiss and hug and share
    kind words—
then we would have handed him the ticket
to a morning of sunshine and fun at school.

I know fights between spouses are normal
and inevitable, Lord,
and bad fights at that.
But this morning my husband and I neglected a key
        element
of a healthy disagreement—
an open, loving resolution for our child to see.
Our child's health, happiness, and personality,
his relationships with friends and family,
his self-image and potential for success at school,
his outlook on life and outlook on love—
all these aspects of his personhood are forming now,
during his childhood,
and his daddy and I are their primary influences.
Dear God, bless our marriage with love and forgiveness.
Help us to respect and support each other
so that we can provide a warm and secure home
for our impressionable little one.

As my husband and I work together
to build our growing family's home life
and as we tackle the home improvement projects
in our hearts, Lord,
we're well-outfitted with the tools

for peaceful conflict resolution.
Of course we *know* we should use time-outs,
we *know* we should be better listeners,
we *know* we should refrain from defensiveness,
name-calling,
and character assassinations.
But we need your help in the hard task
of using these tools, Lord.
After seeing my child so unhappy today,
I am determined now
to work harder at resolving our marital differences
as swiftly, respectfully, openly,
lovingly, and peacefully as possible.
I want my child's life, my husband's life, and my life
to be filled with as much sunshine as possible, Lord.
Help us build skylights of love and happiness
into our hearts and home.
I know we have a life-long process of home
improvement ahead of us
and with your help, I believe that one day
we'll be the proud possessors of a dream home.

❧

As a Boy and as a Man

In the scramble to get to our baby's doctor's
    appointment
on time this morning, Lord,
I kicked over and spilled the dog's water dish
and I knew I had no choice but to clean up
that large, slippery lake
by the back door before we left,
and as I mopped up the mess and as another two
minutes ticked by
a swearword rolled off my tongue.
I know that curse traveled from my lips faster than a
    jetliner
and directly into my child's little ear,
and I'm sorry, God.
I'm not feeling good about myself today.

Now that I'm a parent,
I'm keenly aware more than ever before
of my shortcomings, Lord.
I wish I could be a better mom for my baby's sake.
I wish that my child could look at me
and always admire what he sees.
You know that I'll have a tough time modeling an
        upbeat attitude
for my child on days when I'm feeling like a total
        grouch.
And you know full well what my other failings are,
        Lord.
Dear God, how can I help my child become a good
        person
when I have a hard time being one some days?

Of course I want only the best
for my child's developing character, Lord.
I pray that over time he'll become
a generous, courageous, fair, honest,
responsible, self-disciplined,
humble and compassionate man.
I pray that my child, as a boy and as a man,
will fight for justice.

I pray that my child will have the wisdom
to do the right thing at decision-making crossroads.
I pray that my child will feel remorse
when he's done something wrong.
I pray that he'll shun illegal behavior
and any behavior that's hurtful to him
or hurtful to others.
I pray that my child will see the positive in situations
so that he'll know greater happiness.
I pray that my child, as a boy and as a man,
will respect *all* people and *all* cultures.
I pray that he'll respect and protect our planet
and that he'll respect himself, his own body, his own
    health,
and you, God.
I pray that my child, as a boy and as a man,
will come to know you, need you, and love you,
    Lord.

Dear God,
please fill my child's life with loving, noble mentors
from our community, church, school, and Scout
    programs—
wherever your ways are rewarded.

Please help both my husband and me
to grow, change, and improve too,
so that we'll be better equipped
to guide our child, as a boy and as a man,
in the direction of light instead of darkness.

The Best Defense

I've begun to look more deeply
into my baby's beautiful eyes lately, Lord,
trying to see what the future holds in store
for this beloved child and for his small family.
But I've gathered no information from my baby's
      eyes, God,
and the unknown is unnerving.
Worries bubble up out of my imagination
as I wonder about our child's future
and I need your help in controlling these fears, Lord.

Dear God,
my gravest worry today about all of my child's
      tomorrows
concerns his safety and well-being.
I often find myself sorrow-stricken
when I watch the nightly news

and learn of the hateful and horrible things
that some people do *to children*.
I'm afraid of accidents, abductions, molestation,
firearms, diseases, and all other dangers that could harm
our child.
I know the more independent and grown-up our child
becomes,
the more contact he'll have with our sometimes scary
world.
I know that our child's teen years—
that time of a young person's search for self—
will be filled with every imaginable temptation
which could cause great harm to his body, mind, and
spirit.
Please, Lord, help me do all I can
to guide and keep my child safe during these years,
then remind me to turn my concerns over to you.
Please continue to protect our child in the years to
come
and to send his personal angel to his aid daily.

Another continuous concern of mine, Lord,
is for the safety and well-being
of this child's beloved mommy and daddy.

This child needs the two of us, Lord,
and will need us for many years.
No one in the world could ever replace
this child's mommy
or this child's daddy.
Please remind us to take good care of ourselves.
Please continue to protect us and preserve us
until our child is capable of setting out safely on
    his own.

Dear Lord, I know I worry a lot;
please ease my fears about our family's future
and remind me daily that praying about my worries
is my best defense against them.

❧

This Gift from Heaven

From the moment he arrived in my life, Lord,
I've fallen more deeply in love with this new little
    person
with the dawn of each new day.
Thank you for every hour that we've shared with our
    baby
during his infancy
and for all the times that we'll have together in the
    years ahead.
Thank you for every joy and challenge to come
as we grow up side by side,
our child growing as a person
and his mother and father growing as parents.
Thank you, God,
for our beautiful child,
this gift from heaven
which is more precious than anything else on earth.